Weekend Warrior

Winning with Essential Oils

HOW TO PREVENT AND RECOVER FROM SPORTS INJURIES IN A NATURAL WAY!

Judy Jehn, RMT
Steven M. Petersen, RMT, CNMT, NCBTMB
Gini Kyle, RMT, ANMT

VISION PUBLISHING, LLC
DENVER, CO

Copyright © 2011 by Judy Jehn

1st Edition, August, 2011

Kathryn Caywood, LLC, Editor

Ann Zielinski, Book Design

International Standard Book Number: ISBN 978-0-9818290-2-9

Library of Congress Control Number: 2011934626

Jehn, Judy

Weekend Warrior Winning with Essential Oils /

Judy Jehn, Steven M. Petersen, Gini Kyle

1. Essential Oils. 2. Aromatherapy. 3. First Aid.

4. Massage & Reflexology.

Printed in USA

VisionPublishingLLC.com

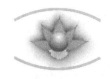

Table of Contents

Put Essential Oils to Work for the Athletes in Your Family

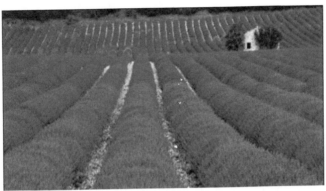

- Understand ways to fuel the body to promote muscle development and reduce incidence of injury

- Learn how to achieve non-drug recovery from muscle, tendon, and ligament damage
  - Learn layering techniques using single oils
  - Find out which oil blend to use for a quick fix
- Discover simple massage techniques to reduce pain and promote lymphatic drainage, hastening recovery for yourself and your family

What are Essential Oils?

- Aromatic liquids of plants, trees, leaves, fruit, and flowers

- Natural oils that have nutritional and therapeutic properties

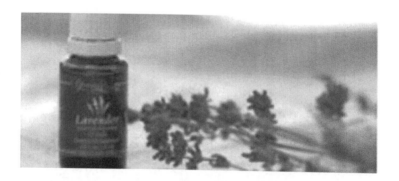

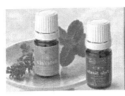

- Essential Oils have the ability to

  - Prevent and relieve the discomforts associated with a wide variety of health problems

  - Reduce stress

  - Lift depression and restore or enhance a sense of well-being

  - Provide revitalizing beauty-care treatments for skin, hair, and body

Phyto = Plant

- **Phytochemical** - the plant's active chemical components (constituents) that account for its medicinal properties
  - Mosby's Medical Dictionary, 8th edition. © 2009, Elsevier.

- **Phytonutrient** and phytochemical are used interchangeably to describe those plant compounds which are thought to have health-enhancing qualities

- More terms: **Phytomedicinal** and **phytotherapy**

Essential Oils
Have the Ability to Influence

Phyto-nutritionally

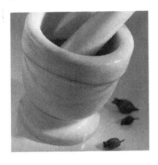

Physiologically

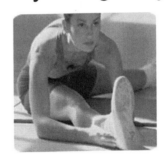

Psychologically

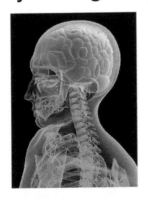

Phyto-nutritionally

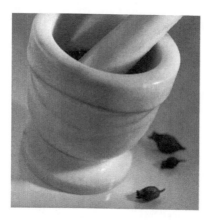

- The human body is made up of proteins - every cell from toenails to hair

- Essential oils are compounds containing amino acids which convert to protein

- When cells are compromised, essential oils start regeneration through the healing properties of amino acids and the increased oxygen to the tissues

Physiologically

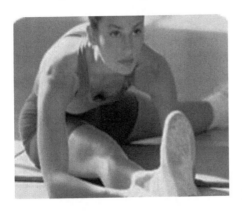

- Essential oils support different areas of the body, for example:
  - Numerous oils from herbs assist in strengthening and realigning the musculoskeletal system
  - Various oils from spices benefit the digestive and immune systems
  - Many oils can break down and detoxify the chemical build up in fatty tissue, potentially clearing DNA

Essential Oils Promote Homeostasis

Psychologically

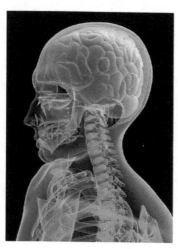

- Through the sense of smell, essential oils soothe the mind and calm the psyche, producing a restorative effect on the emotions

- Some essential oils stimulate the neurotransmitters of the brain

Quality Makes the Difference

- "100% Pure" doesn't mean the same thing in the cosmetic industry

- In the U.S. only 5% real oil needs to be present to be labeled "100% Pure"

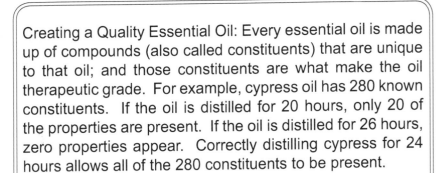

Creating a Quality Essential Oil: Every essential oil is made up of compounds (also called constituents) that are unique to that oil; and those constituents are what make the oil therapeutic grade. For example, cypress oil has 280 known constituents. If the oil is distilled for 20 hours, only 20 of the properties are present. If the oil is distilled for 26 hours, zero properties appear. Correctly distilling cypress for 24 hours allows all of the 280 constituents to be present.

Fingerprinting Methods

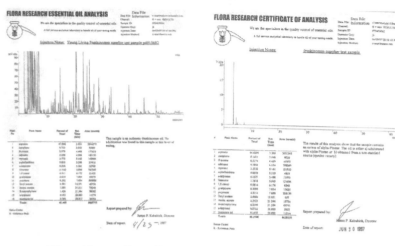

Testing for Purity

- Gas chromatography
- Mass spectroscopy
- Thin layer chromatography
- High performance liquid chromatography

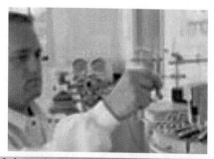

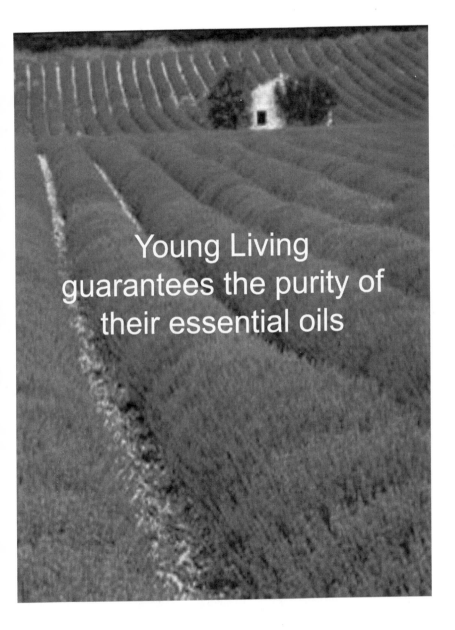

Young Living guarantees the purity of their essential oils

Too Much Too Fast?

- Often the excitement of warmer weather can propel us outside before we've readied ourselves

- A sedentary winter or a free weekend tempts us outdoors without adequate preparation

- Getting in shape before a bike ride or a run isn't even a thought

- Pesky weeds taunt us from the garden

What can we do to prevent injury?

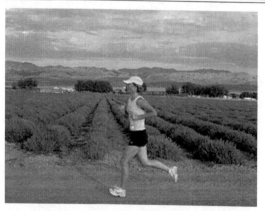

Photo courtesy of Young Living website

FUELING THE BODY TO PROMOTE MUSCLE DEVELOPMENT AND REDUCE INCIDENCE OF INJURY

Work Up to Your Activity and...
Stretch Those Muscles!

Restoring proper length and flexibility to muscles is the biggest contributing factor in pain prevention and reduces acid build-up in the tissues.

Stretching is not a "taffy pull." While exhaling, slowly lengthen the muscle and stop when you feel tension. Muscles will not release if they sense they are at risk, so do not stretch too far. Breathe in while holding the stretch for 30 seconds and then relax the muscle. When the tension has released you can lengthen the muscle further and repeat the breathing process.

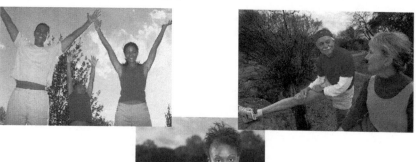

Expanding and Lengthening

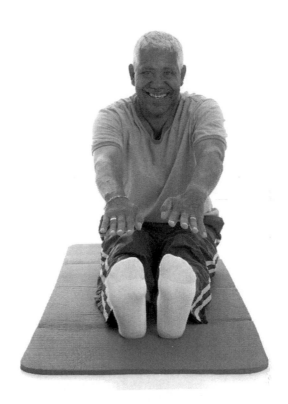

- Keep those muscles limber by drinking enough water and by stretching

- Start slowly and work up to longer runs, hikes, bike rides, gardening

Sports Nutrition

- Carbohydrates - the main nutrient that fuels exercise of a moderate to high intensity

- Fat - fuels low intensity exercise for long periods of time

- Proteins - used to maintain and repair body tissues and are not normally utilized to power muscle activity

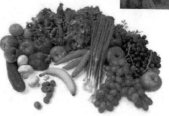

Source: Ask.com

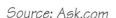
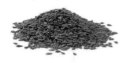

Simple and complex carbs are crucial nutrients and are your body's main source of energy. Fats help your body absorb several essential vitamins to repair your tissues from a workout. Protein (30-35%) – builds everything from muscles and bones to hair and toenails.

Refer to *Fueling Muscles* in the Appendix.

Before Exercise

- Ensure that adequate glycogen storage is available for optimal performance
  - NingXia Red
  - Wolfberry Crisp Bars
  - YL Manna Bars

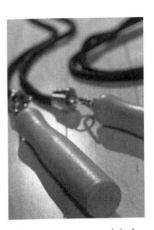

Most other juice drinks contain fructose sugar or high fructose corn syrup, which spikes sugar levels. When your blood sugar levels fluctuate too much, it can wreak havoc inside your body and affect your stamina.

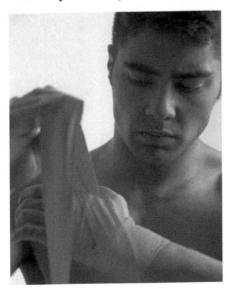

The sugars in NingXia Red are the important polysaccharide sugars with a low glycemic index, which provide endurance.
- Hugo Rodier, MD

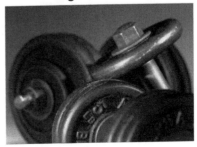

During Exercise

- NingXia Red combined with coconut water for all natural hydration and electrolyte replenishment

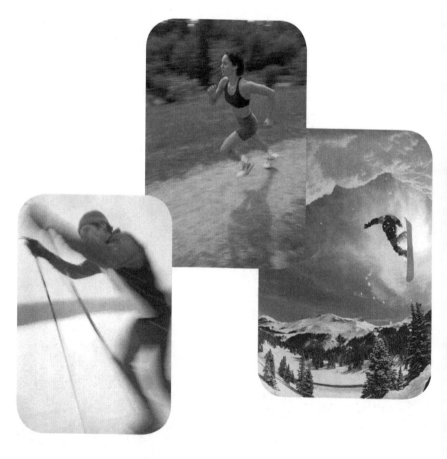

Refer to *Fueling Muscles* in the Appendix.

After Exercise

- Hydration - NingXia Red combined with coconut water
- Carbohydrates plus protein speeds recovery
  - 4:1 carbs to protein
  - that's NingXia Red!
- Pure Protein Complete provides the amino acids necessary to rebuild muscle tissue

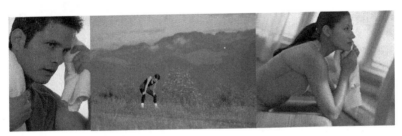

Consuming protein has other important uses after exercise. Protein provides the amino acids necessary to rebuild muscle tissue that is damaged during intense, prolonged exercise. It can also increase the absorption of water from the intestines and improve muscle hydration.

Refer to *Fueling Muscles* in the Appendix. For a handout on Pure Protein Complete, go to www.youngliving.com for the product information page or refer to the Essential Oils Desk Reference.

Pure Protein Complete™

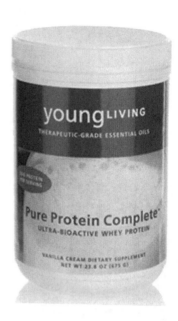

- High in bioactive whey protein, low in carbs, fat, and calories
- Delivers 20 grams of a proprietary whey protein blend supported by a specialized enzyme blend

- Generous amounts of complementary vitamins and minerals

- Sustained protein metabolism and reduced muscle breakdown

- Low glycemic index with no artificial sweeteners

Source: Essential Oils Desk Reference

Power Meal™

- Contains NingXia wolfberries

- Dairy and allergen free

- 20 grams of protein per serving plus a complete vitamin, mineral, and enzyme profile

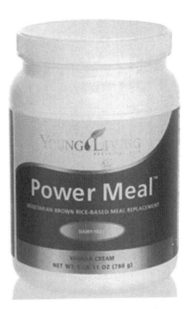

- Rich in calcium, antioxidants and amino acids

- Builds lean body mass with sustained energy release

- Enhances natural detoxification process

- Supports healthy, normal cholesterol levels

Source: Essential Oils Desk Reference

Core Supplements™

- Omega Blue – clinically proven omega-3 fatty acid nutrients and essential oils of German chamomile, myrrh, lemongrass and clove
- Longevity – essential oils of thyme, orange, clove and frankincense to prevent damaging effects of aging, diet and the environment

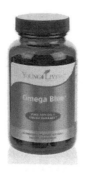
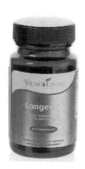
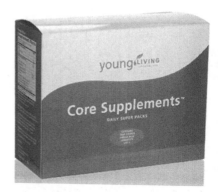

Omega Blue is enteric coated with a special seaweed, to allow assimilation in the small intestine rather than in the stomach; this speeds the absorption without free radical oxidation.

Source: Essential Oils Desk Reference

Core Supplements™

- True Source – uses nutrient-dense super fruits, vegetables, and other plants to deliver the full spectrum of bioactive vitamins, minerals, antioxidants and phytonutrients

- Life 5 – probiotic to build and restore core intestinal health

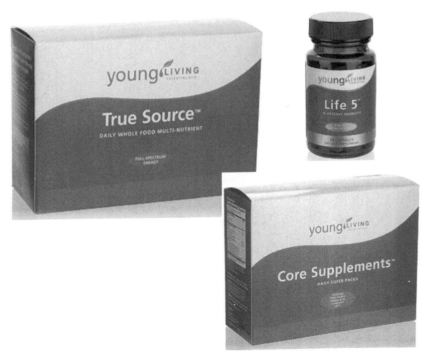

Source: Essential Oils Desk Reference

BLM™
Bones, Ligaments and Muscles

- Supports normal bone and joint health, healthy cell function, and fluid movement

- Combines powerful all-natural ingredients, such as type II collagen, MSM, glucosamine sulfate, and manganese citrate, enhanced with therapeutic-grade essential oils

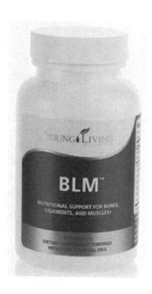

Source: Essential Oils Desk Reference

Enzymes

- Allerzyme - promotes digestion
- Carbozyme – for carbo-loading
- Detoxyme - digestion, detoxification and cleansing
- Essentialzyme - digestion, assimilation of nutrients
- Lipozyme - fat-digesting
- Polyzyme - protein digesting

It's all about absorption!

Before exercise, when you are carbo-loading, try Carbozyme. At the onset of exercise, or during and after, try adding Polyzyme to increase the absorption of your protein intake. If you are doing low intensity exercise for long periods of time, take Lipozyme. Add Allerzyme if your exercise is intense cardio-vascular and outdoors during the summer when everything is in bloom. At bedtime, after an intense day of exercise, take Detoxzyme.

Don't want to take all of those products? Supply your body throughout the day with Essentialzyme.

Source: Essential Oils Desk Reference

Sulfurzyme™

MSM is an organic source of sulfur which is widely utilized by the body in the formation of connective tissue and in the antioxidant glutathione. Sulfur is essential to good health but is easily destroyed by modern food processing methods resulting in widespread deficiencies.

MSM is structurally and functionally important to more than 150 compounds in the body including enzymes, hormones, antibodies and free radical scavengers.

MSM has been used repeatedly for the relief of pain, head trauma, interstitial cystitis, scleroderma, rheumatoid arthritis, osteoarthritis, and Alzheimer's disease.

MSM makes the cell walls flexible and elastic. If the concentration of MSM in the body is too low, the new cells lose some of their necessary flexibility and elasticity.

MSM makes cell walls permeable, allowing water and nutrients to flow freely into cells, and allowing wastes and toxins to properly flow out.

MSM is a powerful detoxifer.

MSM is also nontoxic.

Source: Essential Oils Desk Reference

Sulfurzyme™

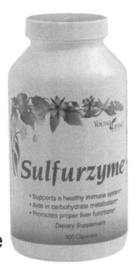

- MSM - dietary sulfur
  - maintains structure of proteins
  - protects/replenishes connections between cells and membranes
  - preserves molecular framework of connective tissue
  - supports the immune system, the liver, circulation and proper intestinal function
  - works to scavenge free radicals

- Wolfberries contain minerals and co-enzymes that support the assimilation and metabolism of sulfur

Source: Essential Oils Desk Reference

More Supplements

- Balance Complete – Superfood meal replacement, high in fiber and protein
- MultiGreens – Boosts vitality and relieves stress
- Inner Defense – Supports all body systems and strengthens gastro-intestinal tract
- Super C – Anti-inflammatory
- MegaCal/SuperCal – Calcium builds bones

Source: Essential Oils Desk Reference

ESSENTIAL OILS SUPPORT NON-DRUG RECOVERY FROM MUSCLE, TENDON, AND LIGAMENT DAMAGE

Notes

What Is Pain?
Why Do We Have It?
Protection Mechanism
"WARNING"

Pain immediately focuses our
attention where we need it to be!!!
It sounds the alarm!!!
"OUCH"

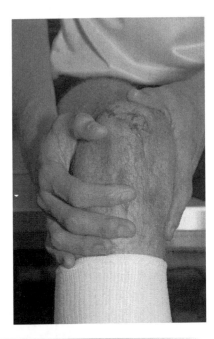

Pain is good. Pain is your
friend. It forces awareness
on a situation that the body
is drawing attention to.

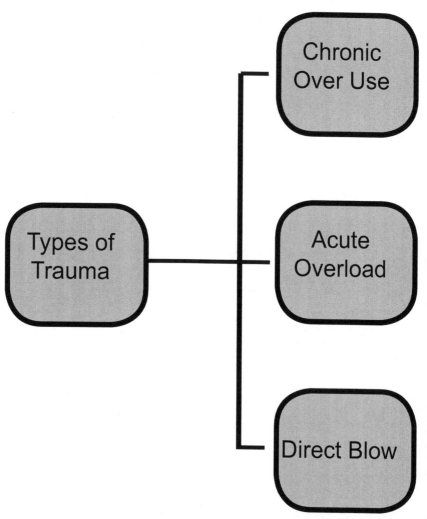

Even though there are three categories of bodily trauma, many injuries are influenced by a combination of these types.

Defining each of the basic types in more detail creates a better understanding of the nature of the trauma, how it occurs, and how they can affect each other.

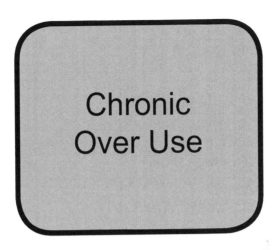

Chronic
Over Use

- Bursitis
- Tendonitis
- Thoracic Outlet Syndrome
- Carpel Tunnel Syndrome
- Degenerative Hip Disease
- Degenerative Disc Disease

Over time, nearly all bodies develop some patterns of over use; however, when they become deeply ingrained, they become painful and can lead to medically diagnosed syndromes.

Habituated Body Patterns

The process of repeated or over use of muscles creates a build up of waste products that accumulate in the muscle tissue. The presence of these waste products triggers the nervous system, which tells the muscle cells to contract in response to the stimulus.

Muscles have three basic responses to this stimulus—splint, protect, and guard—this feels like a tight muscle or a muscle spasm.

A tight muscle creates reduced circulation, resulting in a build up of waste products that cause increased impulses to the nervous system, which in turn creates more muscle contraction.

This process produces habitually contracted muscle patterns in your body. As the muscle pulls on the tendons and ligaments, your body moves out of alignment.

These patterns compress nerves, blood vessels, and joints. Now your body has to compensate for the misalignment by using another area or set of muscles to maintain stability.

The result is a less flexible body that is prone to pain and pre-disposed to injury.

Habituated Body Patterns

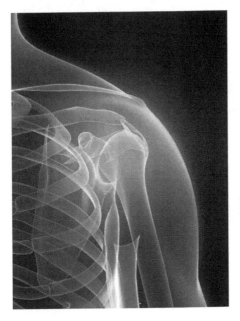

Using muscles repeatedly (chronic over use)

- Causes them to become shorter, tighter, and sore

- Which pulls the bones out of alignment, compressing the joints

- Results in less flexibility, creating a greater chance for trauma or injury (pain)

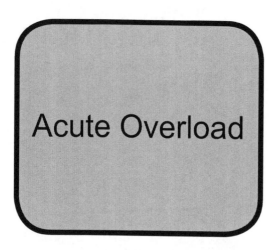

- When muscles suffer a load that is too heavy, too fast, or over extended, trauma can occur

- Strains, pulls, sprains, and breaks can result (micro tears to detachments)

- Habitually tight muscles or misaligned joints are more susceptible to acute overload

Tight muscle fibers are less flexible and tend to tear more easily because they cannot handle the overload. For example, when trying to lift a heavy object and you hurt your back. If your back is tight to start with, it can more easily be injured!

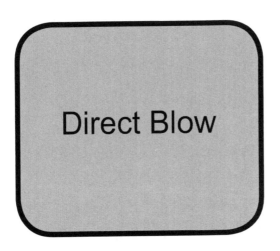

Direct Blow

- An impact from an outside force
- The body hitting something or an object striking the body
- Bruising, swelling, tears, breaks, and abrasions

Severe trauma can cause a pooling of fluid that swells up in the injured area. This produces increased pressure and pain. Applying oils as soon as possible reduces the swelling and results in a quicker recovery.

A direct blow can cause an acute overload as well. A tight body pattern created by chronic over use can suffer an acute overload when struck by a direct blow. This is an example of a combined trauma injury.

Homeostasis

- Human homeostasis refers to the body's ability to physiologically regulate its inner environment to ensure its stability in response to fluctuations in the outside environment and the weather
  - Wikipedia.com

- State of balance in the body

- The body's ability to maintain internal equilibrium by adjusting its physiological processes

When every cell in the body has everything it needs to be happy and healthy, we are in a state of homeostasis. This requires that all systems of the body are functioning and flowing well.

Nutrition plays a crucial part in homeostasis!

Layers of the Body

- Skeletal system

- Nervous system

- Circulatory system

- Lymphatic system

- Muscular system

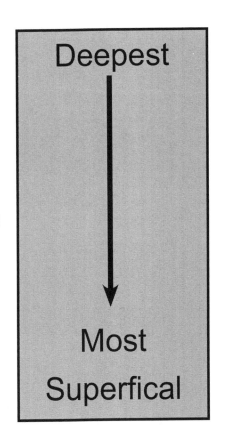

When treating pain, work from the deepest layers to the most superficial layers.

Skeletal System

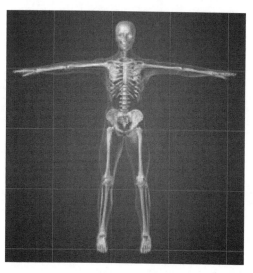

- Bone, ligaments, tendons
- Supports weight in gravity
- Allows movement via joints
- Foundation layer, least flexible

Ligaments and tendons are the densest portion of the connective tissue. The skeleton is the frame for all of our organs and every system of our body - all bodily tissues are literally suspended in gravity, hanging from the skeletal frame and surrounded by water.

When tight and contracted, these connective fibers compress the tissues and joints, constricting movement and restricting the functional flow of the body's systems.

Nervous System

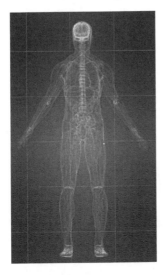

- Neurons, electrical flow
- Communication – relays information
- Central Nervous System is the "master controller"

The nervous system keeps track of everything that is happening in the body and it responds automatically and instantaneously.   It sends conscious commands to the muscular system.

Circulatory System

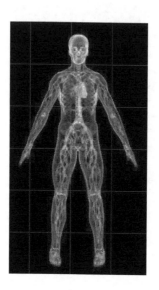

- Blood, plasma flow
- Transports nutrients and removes waste throughout the body
- Arteries, veins, capillaries

The circulatory system is the primary delivery system for nutrients and the waste removal mechanism for unwanted by-products of metabolism.

Lymphatic System

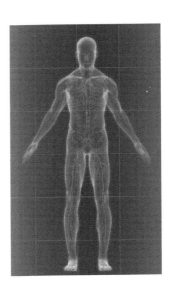

- Eliminates toxic waste and damaged cells
- Brings nutrients, oxygen, and hormones to cells
- Secondary fluid flow

While the cardiovascular system relies on the heart to pump blood, the lymphatic system has no such pump. It relies solely on your body's physical movement to move lymph fluid.

When the lymphatic fluid moves freely, cells are able to get the oxygen and other needed nutrients. The lymphatic system is also responsible for removing metabolic waste, toxins, abnormal cells, bacteria, and viruses from your body.

When a person is relatively inactive, the lymph fluid becomes congested, stagnant, and toxic. A sluggish lymphatic system causes a suppressed immune system and paves the way for many common diseases.

Muscular System

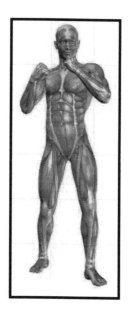

- Muscle, movement, strength
- Moves the bones of the skeleton
- Most superficial

Muscles are the most fibrous of all of the systems. Habitually over-used muscles spasm; the fibers restrict the flow of lymph and blood, compress nerves, and limit skeletal movement.

When this occurs, chronic over use syndromes and injury develop.

This system needs to be flexible!

Common Joint Parts

- Bones
- Ligaments
- Tendons
- Muscle tissue
- Joint capsules
- Cartilage surfaces
- Synovial membrane

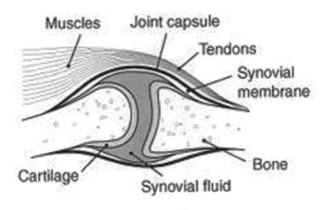

Although muscles are not considered joint parts, they span the joint to allow movement. The focus of this presentation is on the bones, ligaments, tendons and muscles, as they have the greatest effect on the other three joint parts.

Muscle Contraction

- When a muscle contracts, it produces acid waste products that irritate tissues
- Muscles need blood to carry away acid waste and to bring in fresh nutrients

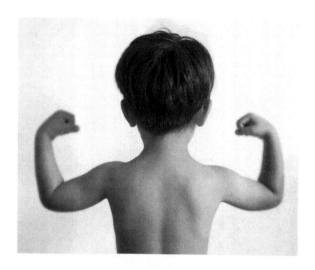

Muscles are what move the joints and are a major contributor to joint pain. The contraction is done by individual muscle cells that pull on the connective fibers in the muscle to move the bones of the joint.

Sensory Input From Joints

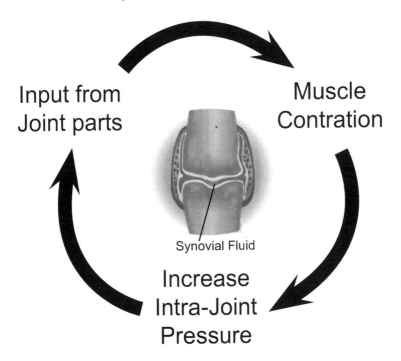

Input from
Joint parts

Muscle
Contration

Synovial Fluid

Increase
Intra-Joint
Pressure

The nervous system is constantly sensing the condition of the joint parts, especially the pressure on the cartilage surfaces. When the cartilage has an increase in pressure, the nervous system contracts the muscles that span the joint in order to protect (immobilize) it. This contracts the joint space and produces pressure on the cartilage that increases the joint's input to the nervous system.

All of the joint parts become inflamed, increasing the sensory input and become trapped in this vicious cycle of chronic pain. Joints in this state are prone to injury. This is the main cause for degenerative joint disease.

Ligaments

- Connect bone to bone
- Keep joints stable
- Ligaments are
  - Mostly fibrous
  - Semi-flexible
  - Areas of low blood supply

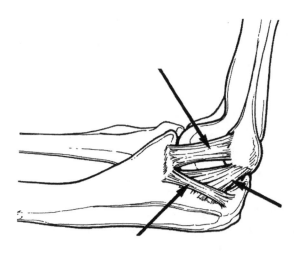

This is an elbow joint showing how the ligaments connect the bones of the upper and lower arm, allowing it to have stable movement.

Tendons

- Connect muscles to bone
- Tendon fibers
  - Are packed tightly together
  - Have a low blood supply

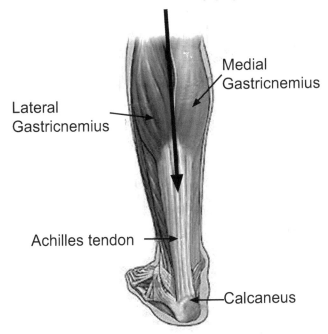

Medial Gastricnemius

Lateral Gastricnemius

Achilles tendon

Calcaneus

More than one muscle of the leg connects into the Achilles' tendon and then merges into the heel bone (calcaneus). Tendon and ligament fibers are densely packed for strength and have little or no capillaries, as they get most of their blood supply from the surrounding tissues.

Tendon and Ligament Fibers Join to the Bone Via the Periosteum

The **periosteum** [per'i·os'tē·əm] is a tough, fibrous vascular membrane that surrounds each bone, except at their extremities.

The periosteum is permeated with the nerves and blood vessels that innervate and nourish underlying bone. The membrane is thick and markedly vascular over young bones but thinner and less vascular in later life. It appears to be the curative agent in the case of bone breakage. Bones that lose periosteum through injury or disease usually scale or die.*

When a muscle has constant or sustained pulling on its attachment to the bone, the periosteum can be separated (pulled away) from the bone, creating slight bleeding (hematoma) and inflammation where it is attached.

The periosteum responds by building calcium on to the tendon or ligament fibers in an effort to strengthen and calm the area. Calcium acts as an anti-inflammatory.

When this occurs, it can form into a sharp point that irritates the muscle tissue. This is how bone spurs are formed. Before a bone spur can be healed, the muscle tension must be released by lengthening the muscle.

* *Source: Mosby's Medical Dictionary, 8th edition. © 2009, Elsevier.*

Tendon and Ligament Fibers Join to the Bone Via the Periosteum

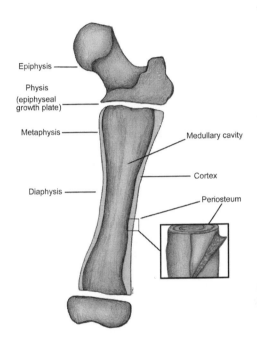

- A fibrous sheath that covers bones
- Contains the blood vessels and nerves that provide nourishment and sensation to the bone

Tendon and Ligament Fibers Join to the Bone Via the Periosteum

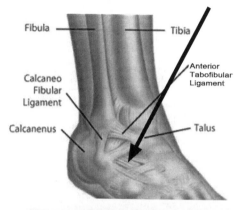

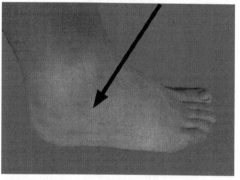

- Increased muscle contraction pulls on the periosteum, causing inflammation

- Most joint injury pain comes from the periosteum, disrupting homeostasis

Blood Supply

- Optimum blood supply to the muscles, ligaments and tendons is vital

- As blood flows through the capillaries, it replenishes nutrients and removes waste products

- This cleans the water in which the cells live and allows the muscles, ligaments and tendons to maintain homeostasis

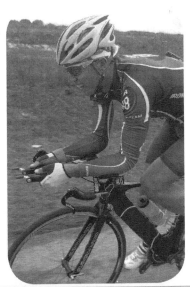

Essential Oils Increase Homeostasis

- Small molecular size increases cellular osmosis

- Lipid soluble based – cell membranes are layers of fats and proteins

- Full of nutrients and elemental constituents that aid healing

The ability of essential oils to increase cellular osmosis allows the cells to function better by eliminating debris and absorbing nutrients with greater ease and speed.

The fat (lipid) soluble bases of essential oils make them highly interactive with the cell membrane.

Essential oils are absorbed directly into the tissues and do not need to pass through the digestive or circulatory systems to benefit the area to which they are applied.

Layering Technique Using Single Oils

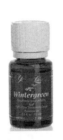
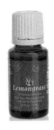
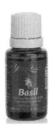
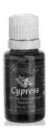

For strains, sprains, and joint trauma, or bruising of the bone

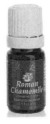
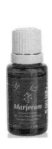
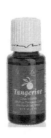
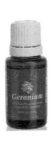
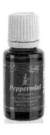

Technique

Attention and Intention

- Essential Oils are a natural tool

- Knowing a tool's function gives it purpose

- Using the right tool with a purpose is intention

- Intention focuses attention

- Focused attention increases results

A nail and a screw are both fasteners. A hammer and a nail are used to quickly fasten wood together, or a screwdriver and a screw for a more secure joining. In each case, there is an expected result based on experience - the intention. Focusing your attention on the intention of your actions creates more actuated results.

Young Living Essential Oils are the highest quality tools and produce excellent results with the right knowledge, focus, and intention.

Technique

Layering Oils

- Apply an oil and wait several minutes for the tissues to absorb it before applying the next oil

- Keeps the molecules of each oil intact and allows them to work purposefully

- Allows for a specific intention for each oil applied

If you apply a base coat of white paint to a wall, it must be dry before applying the red paint if your desire is a red wall. If the white paint is still wet when you apply the red paint, the result is a messy pink wall.

The same principle applies to layering of essential oils when applied to the skin. Allow a minute or two between the layers for the oils to penetrate the skin and absorb into the tissues.

Technique

Wintergreen

Cell membranes have receptor sites that receive supportive nutritious molecules for that particular cell. If the receptor sites are clogged due to petrochemicals or other debris, communication to the cell is blocked, disrupting homeostasis.

Begin the layering protocol with wintergreen, which helps to clean these receptor sites so the cells receive the greatest benefit from the essential oils to be applied in the layering to follow.

Wintergreen has aspirin-like constituents that reduce tenderness in the periosteum, thus lowering the pain stimulus into the nervous system and reducing the chronic pain cycle from the start.

Wintergreen essential oil can feel hot on the skin, so be sure to dilute according to the EDR guidelines.

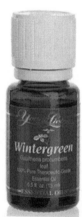

Technique

Wintergreen

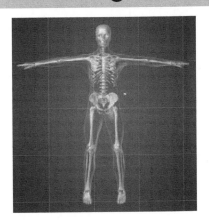

- Analgesic – calms down the pain from the periosteum
- Apply to bone, coating it, and work it in to tolerance, in toward bone

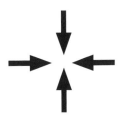

Focus intent on the bones

Source: Essential Oils Desk Reference

Wintergreen and Aspirin
Analgesic Effects

Methyl Salicylate
Comprises 90+% of Wintergreen oil

Acetylsalicylic Acid
Common Aspirin synthetic chemical formulation

Common aspirin has over 80 different synthetic chemical formulations, each having the same chemical structure ($C_9H_8O_4$) and molecular weight. Methyl salicylate, as found in wintergreen essential oil, has an analgesic effect similar to that of cortisone. The formula for wintergreen oil is $C_8H_8O_3$ – nearly identical chemically to aspirin.

A naturally-occurring molecule cannot be patented so aspirin was created. Wintergreen essential oil is safely absorbed directly into the painful area and can begin to work immediately. Aspirin must pass through the digestive system and then be delivered to the area through the circulatory system, thus taking longer to relieve pain. In addition, aspirin may have negative side effects because of the synthetic nature of the compound.

Technique

Lemongrass

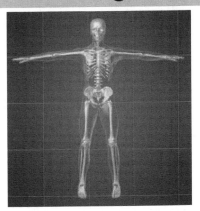

- Supports regeneration of connective tissues

- On top of wintergreen, apply to boney areas of the joints, work it away from the bone towards or into muscle tissue

---

Focus intent on ligaments or muscle attachments

Lemongrass can feel hot to the skin, be sure to dilute according to EDR guidelines.

Source: Essential Oils Desk Reference

Technique

Basil

- Reduces spasms, relaxes and lengthens the muscle fibers

- Start at the tendon (where the muscle connects to the bone), 2-6 drops depending on the muscle size

- Flush towards the heart with gentle, but firm, continuous pressure along the length of the muscle, creating a squeegee like action, slowly pushing the fluids up the muscle

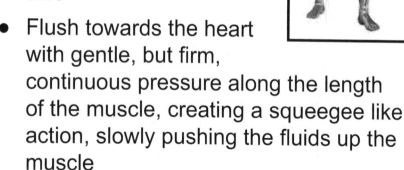

Basil is a powerful muscle antispasmodic, be sure to dilute according to EDR guidelines.

Focus intent on muscles

Source: Essential Oils Desk Reference

Technique

Cypress

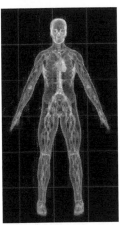

- Increases circulation and promotes lymphatic drainage — discourages fluid retention, strengthens blood capillaries

- Apply 2 - 6 drops directly on the muscle, flush towards the heart

Cypress increases circulation and oxidation to the capillaries, but also helps heal emotional trauma. Soothing and calming, it helps to reduce the feeling of loss, and creates a sense of emotional security, while nurturing and grounding. It absorbs quickly and may need some carrier oil to aid in application.

Dilute oils according to EDR guidelines.

Focus intent on circulation

Optional Technique

Roman Chamomile

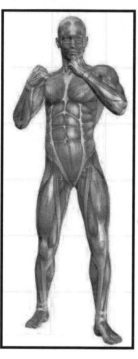

- For stubborn spots where tension still exists

- Allows the muscle cells to release and elongate to their fullest

- Put 1 to 2 drops on the areas that are still tight and work it in toward the heart

Chamomile is also soothing and relaxing; it minimizes anxiety and nervousness.

Dilute oils according to EDR guidelines.

Focus intent on releasing

Source: Essential Oils Desk Reference

Optional Technique

Marjoram

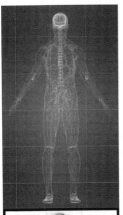

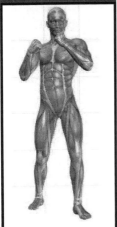

- When nerves are affected, used to warm and open muscle, releasing pressure on nerves
- Muscle-soothing properties help relieve body and joint discomfort after exercise

- Apply 2 - 6 drops directly on the muscle, and flush towards the heart

Marjoram is a general relaxant; it helps soothe the digestive tract and lowers blood pressure.

Dilute oils according to EDR guidelines.

Focus intent on regnerating

Optional Technique

Tangerine

Tangerine is used in the layering technique whenever there is swelling or edema (water retention). It can be dropped on site, then spread or feathered out evenly until mostly absorbed.

Starting at the top (superior) end of the area, use light flushing strokes towards the heart. In one-to-two inch sections, work your way down to the bottom of the area, continuing to flush toward the heart.

It may be necessary to use some carrier oil to assist in gliding over the skin, especially before using long flushing strokes.

Stroke two to three times over the entire length of the area from the bottom to the top, toward the heart to finish up.

Dilute oils according to EDR guidelines.

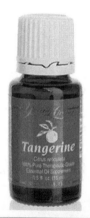

Optional Technique
Tangerine

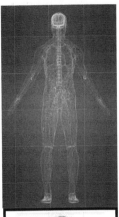
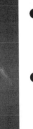
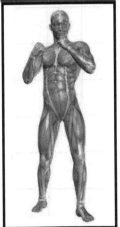

- For lowering fluid retention in tissues
- Reduces spasm, swelling, heat in tissues – hot, "puffy," inflamed
- Drop oil on site, spread or feather out evenly toward the heart
- Photosensitizing – wait several hours before exposing skin to direct sunlight or UV rays

Focus intent on decongesting

Optional Technique

Geranium

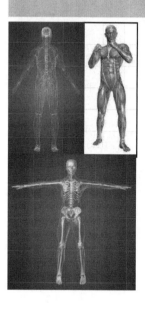

- For bruising or possibility of bruising, use a drop or two on the areas of discoloration

- Lightly rub into tissue, across the bruise first in one direction several times, then several times in the other direction

- Finally, gently flush up towards the heart

Geranium is anti-inflammatory and anti-spasmodic, helping to stop bleeding and improve blood flow. It also may help to relieve nervous tension.

Helichrysum can also be used for bruising.

Dilute oils according to EDR guidelines.

Focus intent on nurturing

Source: Essential Oils Desk Reference

Technique

Peppermint

- Applied last, diluted over the other oils used

- Acts as a catalyst to stimulate the action of the other oils throughout the nervous system

- Spread over the tissue or muscle, follow by light brushing toward the heart using the backs of the finger tips to stimulate the nerves

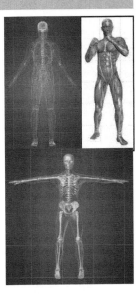

Peppermint is used last to "seal the deal." Because of its strong affinity to soothing the nervous system, it calms and relaxes, thus helping to moderate nervous system responses and "breaking" the Catch-22 effect of tight muscles becoming tighter muscles with nervous stimulants.

Dilute oils according to EDR guidelines.

Focus intent on gently stimulating

Source: Essential Oils Desk Reference

Essential Oil Blends

"A Quick Fix With A Mix"

> # CREATING YOUR WEEKEND WARRIOR FIRST AID KIT

Get the benefits of several oils with one application. And, think about the oil blends that you might want to carry with you on your Weekend Warrior field trip.

Technique

Aroma Siez
Essential Oil Blend

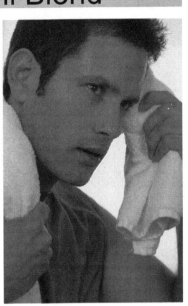

- Use after exercise or at the end of a trying day

- Provides soothing comfort for the head, neck, and tired feet

- Apply to the boney areas and the affected muscles and flush full length of muscle toward the heart

Dilute oils according to EDR guidelines.

Focus intent on muscle relaxation

Source: Essential Oils Desk Reference

Technique

Relieve It

- Reduces inflammation

- For chronic or old areas of aching and deep discomfort

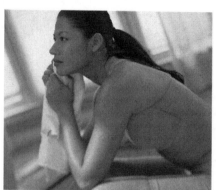

- Apply to the boney areas and the affected muscles and flush full length of muscle toward the heart

Dilute oils according to EDR guidelines.

Focus intent on loosening and relieving

Source: Essential Oils Desk Reference

Technique

PanAway

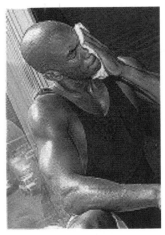

- Relieves bone and joint swelling and discomfort

- Apply to the boney areas, with mild pressure into the dense parts, then mild pressure away from the bone towards ligaments and tendons

- Apply ASAP after injury

Dilute oils according to EDR guidelines.

Focus intent on calming and relieving

Source: Essential Oils Desk Reference

Technique

Deep Relief

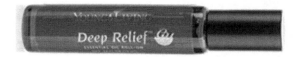

A roll-on is so handy to carry with you and this one relieves muscle soreness and tension, soothes sore joints and ligaments, helps calm stressed nerves, and reduces inflammation.

It contains nine essential oils known for pain relief and anti-inflammatory characteristics.

If applied ASAP after injury, this powerful oil blend may actually help the body to reduce the extent of the injury by bringing healing nourishment to the bone and tissues involved.

Technique

Deep Relief

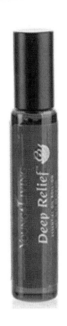

- Use on muscle bellies, joint attachments
- Apply Neat (straight, undiluted)
- Apply to the boney areas, with mild pressure into the dense parts, then mild pressure away from the bone towards ligaments and tendons
- Apply ASAP after injury

Focus intent on relief for the bone, ligaments, tendons, muscles, and nerves

Source: Essential Oils Desk Reference

Ortho Ease Massage Oil

- A soothing massage oil that warms tired or stressed bodies

- An anti-inflammatory and pain-killing complex of vegetable and essential oils

- Ideal for strained, swollen, or torn muscles and ligaments

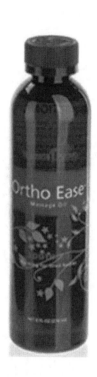

Ortho Sport Massage Oil

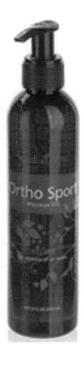

- Stronger version of Ortho Ease

- Designed for both professional and amateur athletes

- Has a higher phenol content, which may produce a greater warming sensation

Regenolone Moisturizing Cream

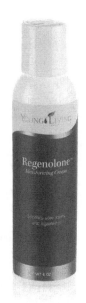

- Muscle and joint pain cream for those suffering severe pain from
  - Inflammation
  - Arthritis
  - Rheumatism
  - Other muscle and joint conditions
- Provides unmatched relief from all types of arthritic, muscle, and skeletal pain

Contains MSM and Pregnenolone.

MSM (methlysulfonylmethane) is an exceptionally bioavailable source of sulfur that restores flexibility to cell membranes and slows the breakdown of cartilage.

MSM has the ability to equalize water pressure inside the cells, which is of considerable benefit for those plagued with bursitis, arthritis, and tendonitis. (See also Sulfurzyme.)

Pregnenolone is the precursor hormone from which the body creates all other sex and adrenal hormones.

Source: Essential Oils Desk Reference

Technique

Cuts, Scrapes and Abrasions

- Use helichrysum or dorado azul to stop the bleeding

- Cleansing the wound

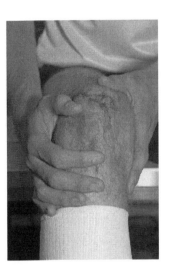

  - Mix Thieves Household Cleaner with water, ratio 1 to 30, in a spray bottle

  - OR, fill an empty Thieves Spray bottle with
    - ½ oz Thieves Fresh Essence Plus Mouthwash
    - ½ oz distilled water

See the Essential Oils Desk Reference for more ideas

Technique

Cuts, Scrapes and Abrasions

- To support wound healing, fill an 8 oz spray bottle with distilled water, add

  - ¼ tsp Thieves Household Cleaner

  - 4-6 drops Purification, *Melaleuca alternifolia* (tea tree), or Melrose

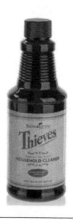

DO NOT USE *Melaleuca alternifolia* (tea tree) or Melrose on puncture wounds—use clove, Thieves, rosemary, or cistus

Cuts, Scrapes and Abrasions

- SCAR-B-GONE Recipe
  - 10 drops helichrysum
  - 6 drops lavender
  - 8 drops lemongrass
  - 4 drops patchouli
  - 5 drops myrrh
  - 1 oz V-6 Enhanced Vegetable Oil Complex

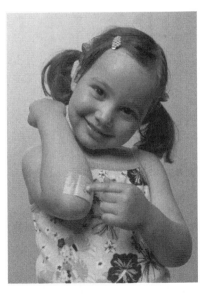

Courtesy of Nancy Sanderson

Severe Trauma Protocol

Everything in this protocol is designed to restrict the extent and swelling of the injury; this results in less pain and a quicker recovery.

For the first 24 to 72 hours, the inflammation will produce its own heat, so use only ice to cool it down. Do not apply ice for more than 10 minutes at a time. Allow the area to re-heat up before applying ice again. Always protect the skin with a cloth before applying the ice.

When the injury is no longer acute, apply the alternating hot and cold therapy to increase circulation. Do not apply heat to inflamed (hot) tissues.

When swelling is still present, always end with ice. This contrast therapy can be used as often as you like and will benefit healing the more it is used.

Contrast therapy promotes circulation because cold creates blood vessel constriction, pushing blood out of the capillaries, and heat creates dilation or opening of the capillaries to allow blood to flow into the area. Alternating cold and hot on an area literally pumps blood through the tissues. Think of it like squeezing and releasing a sponge in water to clean it!

Apply essential oils to the area immediately after icing, while the tissue is still cold. The tissue will be less sensitive when it is cold and as the area warms up the oils penetrate and are absorbed.

Severe Trauma Protocol

> ## Apply essential oils as soon as possible!

- **R** - rest the area by not using it
- **A** - alternate ice and heat
    - ice only for the first 24-72 hours
    - contrast therapy (ice and heat) thereafter
- **C** - compress the swelling area with a wrap
- **E** - elevate the area above the heart

Run a "RACE" Protocol

Before and After

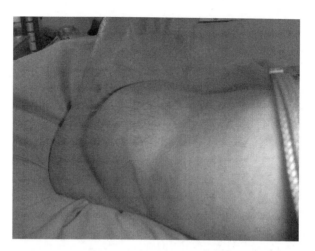

Day 1 – After the first two hours

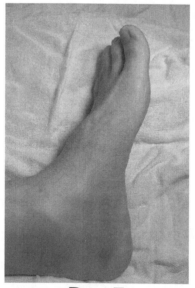

Day 7
Refer to testimony *Sprained Ankle* in the Appendix.

COMBINE ESSENTIAL OILS WITH LYMPHATIC DRAINAGE TECHNIQUES TO HELP REDUCE PAIN AND INFLAMMATION

Lymphatic System

- We have four times more lymphatic fluid than blood

- Lymphatic cells release toxins from the body

- Think of it as the body's garbage collector and eliminator

- Key component in the body's immune system

- Approximately 500-600 lymph nodes are clustered in the body

When injured or when muscles are overused, your lymphatic system can be compromised, affecting proper homeostasis.

Keeping the lymphatic vessels and nodes open and functioning properly may help prevent injury and can significantly assist the healing process.

Lymphatic System

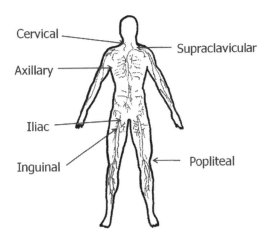

Cervical — Supraclavicular
Axillary
Iliac
Inguinal — Popliteal

Major Lymph Nodes

- Eliminates damaged white and red blood cells, and pre-cancerous cells

- Removes build up of toxic synthetic drugs such as anesthesia and ibuprofen

- Helps bring nutrients, oxygen and hormones to cells

We all have pre-cancerous cells in our body. When not eliminated through the lymphatic system, toxins can collect in areas such as the breast tissue, colon, prostate and uterus.

Moving Lymph

- Muscle contractions and exercise help to move superficial lymph (70-80%)

- Deep respiration helps to pump deep lymph (20-30%)

- Exaggerate arm and leg movements when walking to pump lymph with each step

Aerobic exercises are excellent for pumping lymph - running, bicycling, cross-country skiing. Other exercises include jumping jacks and jumping rope.

Reasons for Manual Lymph Drainage

- Cellular and tissue detoxification

- Improves immune response by increasing T and B cells (the major cellular components of the adaptive immune response)

- Pain relief and reduction of inflammation

- De-stressing

Lymphatic System

- When compromised, the lymphatic system can affect the entire body's normal functioning and healing processes

- Some causes of dysfunction:
  - Inactivity
  - Injury
  - Surgery
  - Inflammation
  - Tight clothes

Technique

Clearing Lymph Nodes

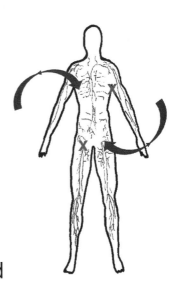

- Apply 2-3 drops lemongrass and/or cypress oil (layering) under right armpit and with left hand gently squeeze 10 times

- Apply oils as marked near right groin (avoiding genitals) and gently push in toward groin 10 times

- Repeat on left arm and groin

Alternate a lymphatic massage with every 3-4 regular massage sessions. Although it is preferable to have lymphatic work performed on you, here are some methods of self-treatment to help keep the lymphatic vessels and nodes open.

Dilute oils according to EDR guidelines

Technique

Moving Lymph

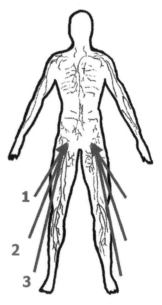

- Layer cypress, lemongrass and/or tangerine on right leg and thigh
- With slow and gentle circular motion, move skin with only enough force to stretch the skin, 8-10 reps per circle
  - Start from upper thigh and use motion toward heart (1)
  - From knee to upper thigh (2)
  - From ankle to upper thigh (3)
- Repeat on left leg (same technique for arms)

Dilute oils according to EDR guidelines

Lymphatic Pump

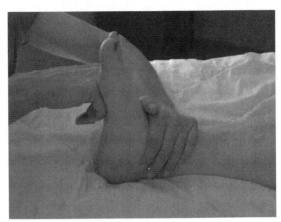

Pushing the foot

- Dilute 2-3 drops each cypress, lemongrass and/or tangerine in V-6 oil and apply to ankles, top and bottom of feet
- Hold right foot with palm of left hand at top of foot/leg joint
- Place right fist on ball of foot
- Push top of foot away from you as far as is comfortable

...continued

Technique ...continued

Lymphatic Pump

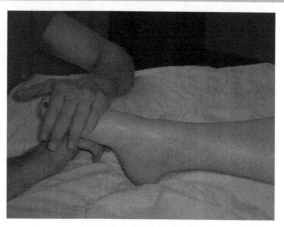

Pulling the foot

- Then slide left hand toward toes while pulling foot as close as possible to table with right fist supporting bottom of foot

- To avoid overextension, verify comfort level

- Return hands to original position

- Pull and push foot using "pumping" motion 10 times for maximum benefit

- Repeat on left foot

Deep Breathing

- De-stresses your body and increases your energy level
- 70% of body toxins are eliminated through breathing
- Releases stored emotions

Seventy percent of body toxins are eliminated through breathing – more than from the bowels! Breath work also raises the blood's alkaline level, a result sought by many health care professionals for slowing down the aging process and retarding disease.

Other substantial benefits of breath work are that it releases stored emotions from your body and accesses the part of the brain that stimulates memory. By learning to breathe consciously, you are able to uncover and release limiting thought patterns from the past.

Technique

Abdominal Breathing

- "Jump start" the lymphatic system that may have been compromised by surgery or injury

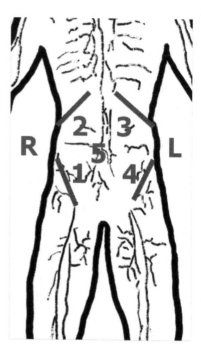

- Important for circulation and muscle tone

- Calming and relaxing when stressed

- Helps to train breathing from diaphragm vs. from neck muscles

See Appendix for details

RELAX AND BREATHE
AAAHHH!!!

Appendix A Fueling Muscles

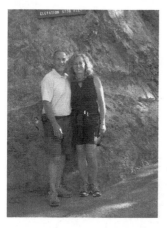

Michael and I desire to stay active as we jump in fully to the second half of our lives! There are many people like me (Connie) who just want to stay active and feel energy. There are others who continue to train on a more athlete status like Michael. Either way consumer choices make a difference in the outcome of your own fitness goal.

Whatever type of person you are, an interesting piece of fitness education is that the <u>University of Texas and St. Cloud State University (MN)</u> shared studies about the importance of a 4 to 1 ratio in drinks (carbohydrates to protein).

The studies stated that the 4:1 ratio is ideal for rehydrating and re-supplying muscle energy stores during exercise. <u>A person's ability to maintain physical intensity is impacted by how you restore fluids and replenish muscle carbohydrate stores while cycling.</u> "During" is the key word. Research showed that the addition of protein improved the muscle's fuel efficiency because it speeds up the carbohydrate uptake and therefore, spared muscle glycogen.

The 4-1 ratio of carb to protein **combined with antioxidants** doubled muscle glycogen levels after exercise. That improved endurance capacity 55% for the next workout. This is why Red caught our attention—and the results of

Appendix A Fueling Muscles

improved endurance proved true but we discovered many additional benefits happened with the NINGXIA RED.

We have found YL's Red and Pure Protein Complete, a bioactive whey protein, are excellent choices for athletes and people who want the endurance to stay active.

a. Red is valuable because it is an excellent nutritive antioxidant drink for sustained energy but it also has the approximate 4:1 ratio. Improved endurance is just one of the benefits we felt. We also experienced the recovery improvements when taking Red.

It is a nutrient dense source. The synergistic effects from the essential oils of lemon and orange cause increased benefits for the body. Plus, we like that it is a beneficial "wholefood" antioxidant. Most of your other juices contain fructose sugar or high fructose corn syrup which spikes your sugar levels. The sugars in Red are the important polysaccharide sugars (Hugo Rodier, M.D). Red has a low glycemic index.

Distance athletes can mix Red with water that contains higher sodium/electrolyte content for those hot, longer endurance challenges. Some athletes mix NINGXIA RED with Gatorade. For normal exercise, we either drink 4 oz straight or with regular water depending on activity. On hot days for longer distance bike rides, I personally like to mix NINGXIA RED with my own homemade lemonade (organic lemon juice, tangerine oil and agave).

Appendix A Fueling Muscles

b. Young Living's Pure Protein Complete is a QUALITY bioactive whey protein. Both Michael and I value this one and it TASTES GREAT. Whey proteins are not the same. There is a big difference in the quality of whey protein products on the market.

American College of Sports Medicine studies say that people who exercise several times a week may not be getting enough protein. Just 30 minutes of aerobic exercise 3 times a week raises the body's need for protein by as much as 25%.

Decide your protein need by dividing your body weight by two. That is your grams in protein. Drink lots of water because it helps wash out the metabolic waste that protein conversion naturally produces. You develop LEAN muscle with proper amounts of protein.

So if you are serious about getting in shape, improving energy and endurance, or just graceful aging, consider a quality fitness nutritional support like Red and a good source of protein like the YL Pure Protein Complete.

Patrick Quillin, PhD., Director of Nutrition for Cancer Treatment Centers of America, says that **life is a continuous balancing act between oxidative processes (pro-oxidants) and protective forces (antioxidants).**

Appendix A Fueling Muscles

We want to fully oxygenate the tissue which generates pro-oxidants, but we then want to protect healthy tissue from excess oxidative destruction using antioxidants. **He views antioxidants as the sacrificial substances to be destroyed in lieu of body tissue**.

Red and Longevity Softgels provide powerful antioxidants. Clove is your highest natural antioxidant on earth—key ingredient in Longevity Softgels. Oil-enhanced nutrition will always give increased benefits. (Order "I Just Know They Work", a recorded webinar and script book from www.bioscentsible.com to hear an accurate and reliable explanation why that is).

Don't forget the importance of enzymes for enhancing fitness. (Michael loves Essentialzyme, a multiple enzyme, and Life 5 Probiotic products from YL.) For those who want to enhance fitness....he knows proper digestion and gut health is one key to endurance. (Michael is a former IronMan Triathlete and personal trainer.)

Try these products for 90 days. It has made a big difference for enhancing fitness and sustaining energy in our lives. I know it will for you too!

Connie McDanel

These statements have not been evaluated by the FDA. Information provided here is for educational use only. It is not for diagnostic or prescriptive use or to be construed as instruction on how to cure or treat any condition, illness or disease. If you have a health challenge, see the health care professional of your choice.

Appendix B Sprained Ankle

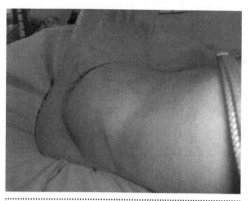

Day 1 – After the first two hours

While jumping over a fence, I suffered a third degree sprain of my left ankle. Luckily, I had PanAway, tangerine, and Believe in my car, so I applied them immediately, which helped reduce the pain enough so that I could stop at the store for ice.

Because my ankle was very swollen and hot, I began using ice on and off. Ice slows down the metabolic process; it stops the swelling and acts as an anesthetic. This was the start of the contrast therapy. I used a towel to protect the skin and placed a bag of ice on the hot area cooling it for 10 minutes; then removed the ice and allowed it to heat back up. This alternating cold and hot helped to increase circulation in a nicely controlled manner.

After removing the ice, I applied the oils of PanAway (a lot at first), wintergreen, tangerine, geranium, lemongrass, Idaho tansy, and Believe (for emotional support). I alternated, using some oils one time and then others the next, getting a broad spectrum of constituents!

Appendix B Sprained Ankle

I applied the oils directly after removing the ice, since the cold decreases the sensation and the area is able to receive light stimulation when gently rubbing in the oils. This initiates the increased circulation and distributes the oils into the area as the tissue begins to warm up.

The next few days were spent doing contrast therapy with ice massage instead of the ice bag. Ice massage is done by taking an ice cube* and rubbing the most swollen and painful areas, using a towel under the ankle to catch the water from the melting ice. Ice massage is very effective for acute conditions and I wanted the ice right where it was needed. I used the same timing, 10 minutes over an area, or until a cold ache was present, then moving the ice massage to another spot. I applied oils after the ice portion of the contrast therapy, at least every hour or so.

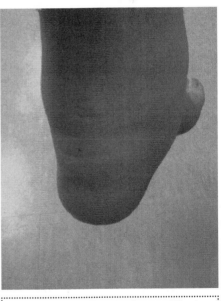

Day 2 – Posterior ankle

* Another method is to freeze water in a paper cup. Use the cup to apply ice massage, tearing away the paper as the ice melts.

Appendix B Sprained Ankle

As the swelling started to go down, I used Regenolone and increased the use of it as the time passed. In the first week, I did not use cypress or peppermint; rather, I chose the oils that promoted reduction of the hematoma (bruising).

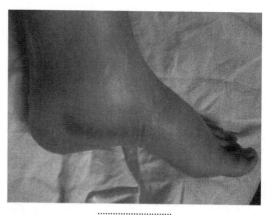

Day 3

At this point, I had wrapped my ankle with an ACE bandage for support and to help reduce the swelling. I had to take the wrap off my ankle to do the contrast therapy and oil application, but wrapped it again when finished.

Sometimes I elevated my ankle for hours, unwrapped, while doing this protocol. Having the wrap off allowed the circulation to flow freely with no increase in swelling or heat while doing the treatment. It felt great to have it off.

Whenever I was trying to move about or sleep, I splinted the ankle (under the wrap) in order to prevent reinjuring the area.

During my recovery time, I never applied any heat to the area at all. The inflamed area was generating significant heat during the healing process; it would throb and become hot all by itself. I tried to prevent this from occurring by using

Appendix B Sprained Ankle

the protocol stated above. If the area generated heat, I knew I was past due for an ice treatment.

Having great belief in the healing power of my body was a big part of my intention. Intention alone did not heal me. I supplied rest, nutrition, oils, supplements, and attention in the form of action.

My pain got my attention. I used knowledge-based actions with consistency and received wonderful healing as a result.

Steven M. Petersen

Day 5

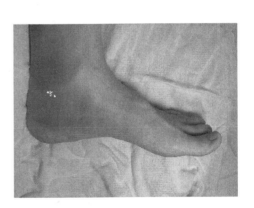

These statements have not been evaluated by the FDA. Information provided here is for educational use only. It is not for diagnostic or prescriptive use or to be construed as instruction on how to cure or treat any condition, illness or disease. If you have a health challenge, see the health care professional of your choice.

Appendix C
Abdominal Breathing Technique

Abdominal Breathing is important for circulation and muscle tone. Use this technique when stressed to impart a feeling of calm and relaxation; or, to "jump start" the lymphatic system that may have been compromised by surgery or injury

1st hand positions, lying on your back:

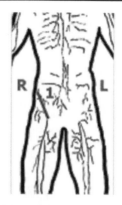

- Place flat right hand just inside the top of the right hip bone (iliac crest) – parallel to the bone
- Place left hand over right
- Push belly out with slow inhalation and, with slight resistance, allow your hands to rise with the belly
- Gently push in with hands on slow exhalation, not deep enough to be uncomfortable

Appendix C
Abdominal Breathing Technique

2nd hand positions – switch hands

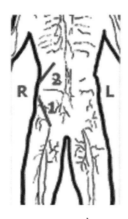

- Place flat left hand under lower right rib (by diaphragm)
- Place right hand over left
- Push belly out with slow inhalation and allow your hands to rise with the belly
- Gently push in with hands on slow exhalation, not deep enough to be uncomfortable

Appendix C
Abdominal Breathing Technique

3rd hand positions – switch hands

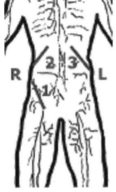

- Place flat right hand under lower left rib (by diaphragm)
- Place left hand over right
- Push belly out with slow inhalation and allow your hands to rise with the belly
- Gently push in with hands on slow exhalation

4th hand positions – switch hands

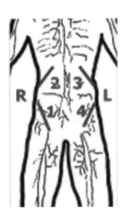

- Place flat left hand just inside the top of the left hip bone (iliac crest) – parallel to the bone
- Place right hand over left
- Push belly out with slow inhalation and allow your hands to rise with the belly
- Gently push in with hands on slow exhalation

Appendix C
Abdominal Breathing Technique

5th hand positions

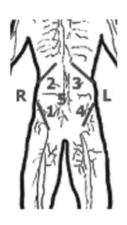

- Place hands over belly button, either hand on top
- Push belly out with slow inhalation and allow your hands to rise with the belly
- Gently push in with hands on slow exhalation

Note: This five position routine may be repeated 2-3 more times for ultimate de-stressing.

Bibliography and Webliography

123RF, Royalty Free Stock Photos, http//www.123rf.com

Essential Oils Desk Reference, 5th ed., Life Science Publishing, 2011, www.LifeSciencePublishers.com

Jehn, Judy, RMT. Aromatherapy for the Soul—Spiritual and Emotional Empowerment with Essential Oils, Vision Publishing, LLC, Denver, CO, 2008

McDanel, Connie and Michael, various presentations and newsletters

MedicineNet.com, 1999

Mosby's Medical Dictionary, 8th edition. © 2009, Elsevier, www.medterms.com

Stewart, David. Healing Oils of the Bible, CARE Publications, Marble Hill, MO, 2003

Young, D. Gary. Essential Oils Integrative Medical Guide, Essential Science Publishing, USA, 2003

Young, D. Gary. Aromatherapy: The Essential Beginning, 2nd ed. Essential Science Publishing, Orem, UT, 1996

Index

Technique Index